If Known What I Know Now

A Guide to
Spiritual and
Practical
application
for Health and
Wellness

DR. LORENZO LEE

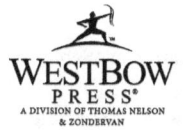

WESTBOW
PRESS®
A DIVISION OF THOMAS NELSON
& ZONDERVAN

WestBow Press books may be ordered through booksellers or by contacting:

WestBow Press
A Division of Thomas Nelson & Zondervan
1663 Liberty Drive
Bloomington, IN 47403
www.westbowpress.com
1 (866) 928-1240

Scripture taken from the King James Version of the Bible.

ISBN: 978-1-5127-5224-3 (sc)
ISBN: 978-1-5127-7166-4 (e)

Library of Congress Control Number: 2016912543

Print information available on the last page.

WestBow Press rev. date: 6/2/2017

Acknowledgements

I would like to give thanks to the almighty one, God, who is first in my life and inspired me to bring this book to life.

I also give thanks to my family; my wife Ra'Shelle for her understanding of the heart felt burden that was placed upon me to write this book. She knows how much I love our Christian brothers and sisters.

Finally, I would like to thank Dr. J.L.Johnson PHD, LNC for his invaluable work in the area of herbal healthcare, which is detailed in his book titled "Common Sense Health"

Introduction: Coming from the Heart

In my introduction to try to let Christians know that we shouldn't sit back and let society dictate what we should know to do. God has given us the sense of being responsible for our life. When God saved us from our negative way of living, he saved us so that we would begin to practice those things of the spiritual life.

I find it ironic in comparison; the things of the Bible, in reference to our spiritual life, the things we should and shouldn't do. They are instructions on once we have been saved and confess the understanding of what the Lord did when he died and rose again, giving us the opportunity or right to have eternal life.

All of those things are well and good in our Christian life but still I thought – as I was sitting and thinking about all of the guidelines the Bible has given Christians – such as "study to shew thyself approved unto God, a workman that needeth not be ashamed, rightly dividing the word of truth"-2 Timothy 2:15, a reference to making sure that you understand what the scriptures are actually telling you about your practical life.

As you go around living among the people of the world, it is important that the things that you used to do you don't do anymore, but instead, observe those things that the scriptures have indicated for us to do. Live according to the scriptures. However, in studying, reading and practicing, the things that you read or the things that the preacher has preached are important, as well as, the things that man has provided for us to live by as we go through life.

What I mean is that the foods we eat and the drugs we take are all important to us as Christians. And yes, the Bible indicates that if something happens or "if we are not feeling well or are sick, to call for the elders of the church-James 5:14, and the prayer of faith would move to hasten us to recovery; but I look beyond just the effort of the Bible in reference to how Christians overcome illness in the body.

We have those things on a spiritual level which may be why our Christians are ill and become so sick that they cannot perform. There are areas in the Bible where it talks about taking the Lord's Supper, which tells us not to take it unworthily. For if you do take it unworthily, you are subject to having a feeble or weak body and some sleep-I Corinthians 11:27-29.

We are not disregarding the scripture in that area but I have looked at some of the things that we can help. We can exhibit control in our everyday walk with the Lord. There is a lot of temptation in the world on a spiritual level on spiritual living; however, there is also a lot of temptation regarding what we eat. There are commercials on television advertising new burgers and fast foods that are geared for our consumption or to motivate us to buy these products.

The same way that we in the spiritual can't seem to stay away from sin and temptation, the guidelines of the Bible tells us to fast and pray, read your scriptures; "man shall not live by bread alone but by every word that proceeds out of the mouth of God" Matthew 4:4, so we must adhere to those teachings. It takes it a little further; we have to be conscious of where we are and what country we are in, as well as some of the records must be more visual as it relates to the things that we put inside our bodies.

Yet as Christians, I am troubled that we trust the "governing system" such as the Food and Drug Administration (FDA), which governs as manufacturers produce these foods as well as what is put into these foods for our consumption. But the records show that the foods we eat here in the U.S. is, as we have found through many years of studying and reading, not necessarily good for us.

The additives and preservatives are not good for the body. As a matter of fact, there are a lot of these things added to our food that makes the body sick if you consume large portions of it. Knowing that these things are causing harm to our bodies, we must make different choices.

Think about back in the days when cigarettes were allowed for commercialization. People got hooked on smoking and it was determined that the nicotine caused certain types of illness. We must realize that these things are all based on lies that the system is giving to the public just to make more money which is called capitalism.

This book that I am bringing to light is to allow our Christians to be aware of their surroundings and not eat and drink everything that is put before them. Be aware that everything that looks good isn't good for you. I have found out, through my lecturing and teaching over the years, that a lot of our Christians are relying on the "I'll pray over it and that will make it ok" syndrome. Yes, we bless our food because we are thankful that we have food, however, once knowledge is imparted to us, we must govern ourselves accordingly. The same as when we were in the world and first received knowledge of salvation, we changed our way of thinking and behavior. We read the scriptures regarding a better life, a spiritual life, a holy life and we took heed to what the spirit of God is telling us. That's when God changes our life…. The same principle applies here.

Once you hear that the foods you are consuming are bad for you or leading you astray, I recommend a change in your diet. We must realize that Satan comes in many forms such as the angel of light-2 Corinthians 11:14. The United States' practice of allowing companies to distribute foods for our consumption without considering the consequences of collateral damage, which is us the general public. If you eat so much of this food, it will begin to affect your body negatively by clogging your arteries; as well as many cancers are also linked to the foods we eat now.

Research and testing has proven that our Christians are not playing on a level field as it relates to the foods we eat and drink. We just can't continue to blindly eat and drink everything that is presented as "good for us" and, research has shown that those things are not good for you and will make you sick. So what I am saying here, in this introduction, after many years of study, is that I have watched and understood, from different perspectives, how we have been underserved as it relates to food and drugs.

I was privileged to have a close friend who was a medical doctor. I sat under his tutoring for many years observing and understanding how the system works, and of course after he completed medical school he took an oath regarding what drugs he needs to prescribe for an individual to help him/her to recover. In my observation, I watched countless representatives from pharmaceutical companies come into his office, like a revolving door, offering new drugs. These drugs entered the market for practicing physicians to give to unsuspecting patients to take these drugs and, hopefully, it would cure, or at the very least, make the patient feel better. It is like being a guinea pig. As a new drug is developed, it is given to the patient to see if it is compatible to what ails the patient.

We have all been in the doctor's office and he or she tells you to try this drug or that drug, since they have free samples, and ask that you let them know how you feel when you take the drug. If you feel okay, and the drug helps what ails you, you probably will accept a prescription for that particular drug.

It is this type of activity that I have observed over the years with our physicians, and a lot of times these drugs will have tremendous side effects on an individual. However, the system has changed from previous years regarding the disclosure required by pharmaceutical companies to advise the public of these side effects before they take these drugs. Most times the doctors prescribe these medicines and you take them without questions or challenges, and sometimes they cause serious illness and even death.

Don't misunderstand what I am saying here; there is a place for these chemical drugs, as they can be used to stabilize the body, but not to cure it. For the body to heal itself we, Christians, must take a different approach as it relates to sickness; such as diabetes, heart disease, high blood pressure and cancers.

I am trying to alert Christians to the fact that there is a better way for us to be able to not only be professional in our everyday life but to be professional in our spiritual life also – we can thrive! God wants us to prosper and to be in good health as our soul prospers-3 John 1:2. However, this is not the case often times through Christendom.

As I travel around the United States, I witness sickness amongst our leaders – from Bishops to lay people – who are sick and can't make it to church nor do any work for the Lord due to health constraints caused by the foods we eat and the drugs we take. Once we have come to the knowledge of the truth, we want to change what we eat and drink along with the drugs that we allow in our bodies. Certain sugars are even devastating to the body, such as substitute sweeteners and processed white sugars which attributes to diabetes. We should, instead, discipline ourselves to eat more fresh vegetables and fruits along with organic foods for better health.

The teaching in this book is here for you to have knowledge. For the Bible says, "My people parish for they lack knowledge, for they reject knowledge" Hosea 4:6. Once you receive knowledge don't reject it. Instead, ask God for strength to change your habits. Those are the prayers that are important. Don't be afraid to change your old way of thinking. Awareness and knowledge are the keys to change!

Why are Christians sick: For you to know you need to know

I am saddened.

It frustrates me to see our Christian brothers and sisters, when the pastor ask if any among you are sick to come up for prayer, that often times, it's the same people who come up to be delivered from whatever illness they may have. What happens next is: that brother or sister ends up in the hospital or needing surgery. I realize that the Bible says, plainly, "If any among you are sick call the elders of the church and they will pray the prayer of faith and deliverance "James 5:14. The scripture also says, "I wish above all that you prosper and be in health as your soul prospers"3 John 1:2.

Is it possible that these Christians have an underlying problem that is un-known to them because of the lack of knowledge? There is one cliché that says, "If you know better you will do better". What I am simply saying is that our Christians are eating things that are harmful to the body. There is a simple thing our Christians can do to help their body heal itself. When fasting and praying, ask God for strength and will power to stay away from the foods that make their bodies sick.

I know for a fact that our Christians are aware that they are eating things that are harmful to their bodies as they make statements like, "I know this is going to raise my blood pressure but I am going to eat it anyway".

Christians, do you know that in the U.S. our foods contain additives that are very harmful to the body? The pharmaceutical drugs are processed with so many chemicals, that the side effects from taking these drugs do more harm than good for whatever is ailing you. They are so harmful that these drugs can actually kill you before the illness, which you were taking them for, does.

In this book there are some statistics and practical things your need to be aware of. Are you drinking a lot of water but still thirst? This is a problem for many Christians. The medical experts will not tell you that drinking too much water will weaken your kidney's ability to function. I was a victim of drinking too much water and still was suffering from dehydration and my skin was parched and dry. One thing I discovered was to drink a PH balanced water with electrolytes because it is naturally alkaline. Another bad habit is consuming processed white sugar. This should be replaced with cane raw sugar.

Soda, sweet teas, juices from the supermarket, dairy products such as cow milk, should be replaced with rice, almond or soy milk. Too much red meat, and fats that come from animals, need to be replaced with fresh vegetables and fruits. Eating more organic items, and whole grains are better for our Christians.

Can Christians be so spiritual that they would ignore the statistics showing that what they are eating could make them sick or even kill them? Diabetes, heart disease and cancer are all products of eating the wrong things. Some will say, "if I pray over my food, it will be okay", but again, the scripture says, "My people are destroyed for they lack knowledge, for they reject knowledge" Hosea 4:6. The scripture says to "study to show thyself approved, and a workman need not be ashamed in dividing the word of truth" 2 Timothy 2:15.

As Christians we need to be vigilant in everything in life. Satan does not only try to tempt us with sexual sins, however, he comes to tempt us with other things that we love such as eating, drinking, gossiping, etc. Praying over your food is not enough. That is why the Lord placed on my heart to give His people this knowledge through a book. He told me to go all over to share this knowledge with my people.

Here are more statistics:

U.S. Foods Chockfull of Ingredients Banned in Other Countries

More than, 3,000 food additives – preservatives, flavorings, colors and other ingredients – are added to U.S. foods. Many have been deemed too harmful to use in other countries.

The Terrifying Side Effects of Prescription Drugs

The side effects of prescription medication can be horrific. Is it really worth taking medication if the cure is worse than the disease?

Dr. Mercola's Comments:

Every year, more than 2 million Americans suffer from serious adverse drug reactions. These reactions cause about 100,000 deaths per year.

Drug Side Effects:

Some drugs can't help but trigger side effects because of their chemical structure.

Drug Side Effects: The FDA's Role

Before a drug can come on the market it must be approved by the FDA. This proof comes from testing of the drug, first in animals and then in humans. Once the basic questions of safety and efficacy are settled, the FDA will approve the drug if it deems that its benefits outweigh its risks.

Processed Foods Depend on Additives

When foods are processed, not only are valuable nutrients lost and fibers removed, but the textures and natural variation and flavors are also lost. After processing what's left behind is a "pseudo-food" that most people wouldn't want to eat.

So at this point, food manufacturers must add back in the nutrients, flavor, color and texture to processed foods in order to make them palatable, this is why they become loaded with food additives.

Russia Issues Long-Term Ban on U.S. Meat

In related "questionable food" news, Russia recently banned U.S. meat supplies after discovering it contains ractopamine – a beta agonist drug that increases protein synthesis, thereby making the animal more muscular. This reduces that fat content of the meat. As reported by *Pravda*, Russia is the fourth largest importer of U.S. meats, purchasing about $500 million-worth of beef and pork annually.

Effective February 11, Russia will no longer allow U.S. meat imports, stating the ban "is likely to last for a long time."

What's the Simplest Way to Avoid Harmful Food Additives?

Ditch processed foods entirely. (If you live in Europe you may have more options that American, as you may be able to find some processed foods that do not contain any synthetic additives.) About 90 percent of the money Americans spend on food is spent on processed foods, so there is a massive room for improvement in this area for most people.

Americans' Unhealthy Diet

Pizza, hot dogs, chicken wings, sodas and chip dips are all staples of the American diet that can be found at any pre-football game gathering. Loaded with salt.

Sugar

A high sugar consumption can cause weight gain, a growing problem in the United States, where two-thirds of women and three-fourths of men are overweight and more than one-third of all adults are obese.

Family Testimonial

One day my wife became very ill with a fever, which registered over 102 degrees for over one month. After an emergency room visit and many doctors advice on medicine to try, nothing helped to break the fever. Blood test gave the diagnosis that she had inflammation in her blood. So I encouraged her to try Dr. Johnson's special tea. A few hours later the fever began to break and within three days my wife was back to normal – Praise God!

Christians, the following information is what you need to know to be healthy.

Be blessed.

I say to my fellow Christian brothers and sisters, if you want to be well like my wife Ra'Shelle, in addition to reading "If Known What I Know" please read Dr. Johnson's book titled "Common Sense Health" in which he gives the readers valuable insight concerning our health and wellness.

Dr. Johnson's book helps you navigate and solve over 50 major health complaints.

Question?

Does herbs address health concerns such as STD's in our Christian family? The answer is yes.....

I receive calls regarding STD concerns from our Christian family all over the country. A study conducted by Dr. Johnson called "Unified Advanced Herbology" where herbs are used to cleanse, regulate and rejuvenate your body and the body heals itself.

HERBS ARE A BLESSING TO CHRISTIAN FAMILIES

First of all, I've been using herbs for over 15 years and "I FEEL GREAT".

Here are some of the positive effects herbs have had on my body:

- They strengthen my immune system.
- I have a higher level of energy.
- They help control my gout condition.
- They help lower my blood pressure without the use of chemical drugs.

VITAMIN AND MINERALS

Why are vitamins and minerals along with eating more organic foods so important to our Christian family?

Large quantities of foods that have been approved by organizations such as F.D.A. (Food and Drug Administration) have harmful amounts of bad ingredients. What we need are vitamins and minerals to ensure that our body performs at optimum levels.

Dear Christian,

I'm writing this closing concern letter to you because I've heard your plea from the many calls that I have received.

I know, as a representative of Christ, we too suffer in the body as my family was affected by some of the things that you just read. "If Known What I KNOW NOW" IS A GUIDE TO A SPIRITUAL AND PRACTICAL APPLICATION FOR HEALTH AND WELLNESS.

Dr. Johnson's book called "Common Sense Health" talks about health issues and the role that herbs play in the body healing itself. Now I ask all of my beloved Christian brothers and sisters, church leaders as well as pastors, superintendents and some of our bishops to listen very carefully…I have been taking these same herbs for years for my wellness and there has been no side effects experienced using herbs in lieu of chemical drugs. There is a combination of herbs called Daily Three: (Body Healer, GAP Pills and Immuno Force) which cleanse your blood, colon, upper and lower parts of your digestive system also the liver, lungs and pancreas. I personally take these as maintenance for my body to keep it well, I also take a combination of herbs for my prostate to keep it clean every 90 days. These herbs are called "Total Man, Immuno Force and Prostate Pills" along with a special tea for best results. I know a lot of our leaders have and is suffering with arthritis or gout. If you have suffered with this most painful form of arthritis, you know that it's very painful however, the Lord has bless us with the herbal formula called Arpanex C. This formula along with watching my diet has completely solve my gout problem. I also recommend that you stay away from white sugar, sugary drinks, reduce your intake of red meat and shellfish for best results.

I have received calls from our leaders with complaints of the room spinning when they get up in the morning. When they go to the doctor for a checkup, they are given chemical drugs for the spinning in their head which addresses only the symptoms and not the cause. Listen Christians, if you experience vertigo symptoms in the head this usually caused by kidney malfunction. If you suffer with this condition, I advise that you take a special herbal formula made by Dr. Johnson which cleanses, regulates and rejuvenates your kidney. There are many herbal formulas that address issues suffered by our Christian women and men.

In closing, Dr. Johnson's book Common Sense Health answers over 50 complaints that Christians suffer from. My family has been blessed by these herbs in lieu of chemical drugs when attacked by certain ailments within our bodies.

God said in Genesis 1:29-30, "I have given you every herb bearing seed which is upon the face of all the earth and every tree, in which is the fruit of a tree yielding seed; to you it shall be for meat." In other words, God has said that we shall eat the leaves of the trees, fresh vegetables, fresh fruits, beans and peas (meat) and we shall use God's herbs for the healing of our bodies. Do you know that God took the time to put over 200,000 herbs on the earth and another 9,000 in the ocean, all to help our bodies heal itself?

> "Beloved, I wish above all things that thou mayest prosper in all things and be in health, even as thy soul prospers." (3 John 1:2)

> "Is there no balm in Gilead; is there no physician there? Why then is not the health of the daughter of my people recovered?" Jeremiah 8:22

Be Blessed…

GLOSSARY OF SELECTED HERBS
Benefits and Uses

In general use, herbs are any plants used for food, flavoring, medicine, or fragrances for their savory or aromatic properties. Culinary use typically distinguishes herbs from spices. Herbs refers to the leafy green or flowering parts of a plant (either fresh or dried), while spices are produced from other parts of the plant (usually dried), including seeds, berries, bark, roots and fruits.

Herbs have a variety of uses including culinary, medicinal, and in some cases, spiritual. General usage of the term "herb" differs between culinary herbs and medicinal herbs. In medicinal or spiritual use any of the parts of the plant might be considered "herbs," including leaves, roots, flowers, seeds, root bark, inner bark (and cambium), resin and pericarp.[1]

Herbal supplements, sometimes called botanicals, aren't new. Plants have been used for medicinal purposes for thousands of years. However, herbal supplements haven't been subjected to the same scientific scrutiny and aren't as strictly regulated as medications. For example, although makers of herbal supplements must follow good manufacturing practices — to ensure that supplements are processed consistently and meet quality standards — they don't have to get approval from the Food and Drug Administration (FDA) before putting their products on the market.

Yet all herbs — including herbal supplement products labeled as "natural" — can have drug-like effects. Anything strong enough to produce a positive effect, such as lowered cholesterol or improved mood, is also strong enough to carry risk. So it's important to do your homework and investigate potential benefits and side effects of herbal supplements before you buy. And be sure to talk with your doctor, especially if you take medications, have chronic health problems, or are pregnant or breast-feeding.[2]

[1] Source: https://en.wikipedia.org/wiki/Herb

[2] Source: http://www.mayoclinic.org/healthy-lifestyle/nutrition-and-healthy-eating/in-depth/herbal-supplements/art-20046714

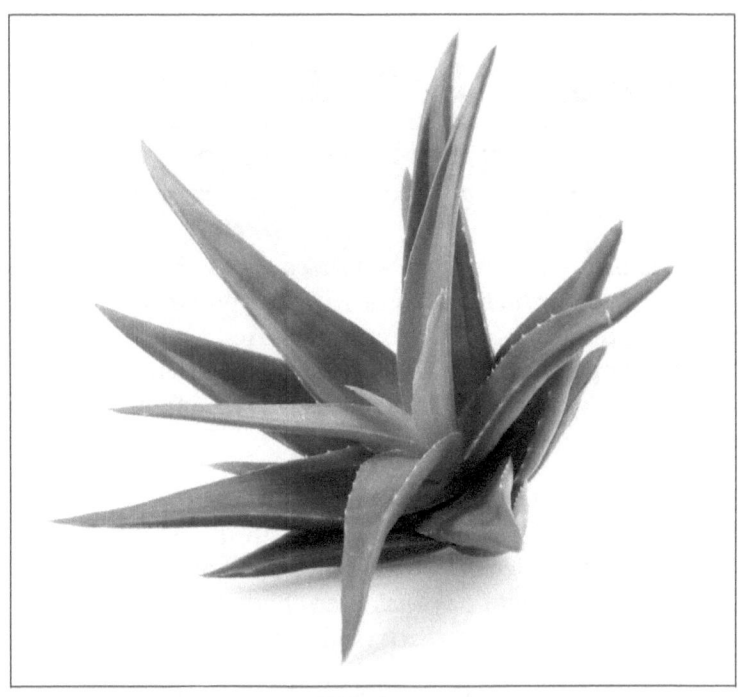

Aloe Vera

The aloe vera plant is considered to be a miracle plant because of its numerous curative and healing benefits. Aloe vera leaves are filled with a gel containing vitamins like A, B1, B2, B3, B6, B12, C and E, and folic acid.

Minerals found in aloe vera juice are copper, iron, sodium, calcium, zinc, potassium, chromium, magnesium and manganese. All these nutrients have tremendous health benefits.

Health experts regard aloe vera as nature's most impressive and versatile herb. This herb is safe to use externally and internally. People across the globe use this herb for treating various health conditions from minor burns to cancer.

Aloe vera is full of antioxidants, which are natural immune enhancers that help combat free radicals in the body. Free radicals are unstable compounds that are bad for your health and contribute to the aging process.

Drinking aloe vera juice regularly gives the body a regular supply of antioxidants, which can boost and enhance the immune system.

Source: http://www.top10homeremedies.com/kitchen-ingredients/10-health-benefits-of-aloe-vera.html

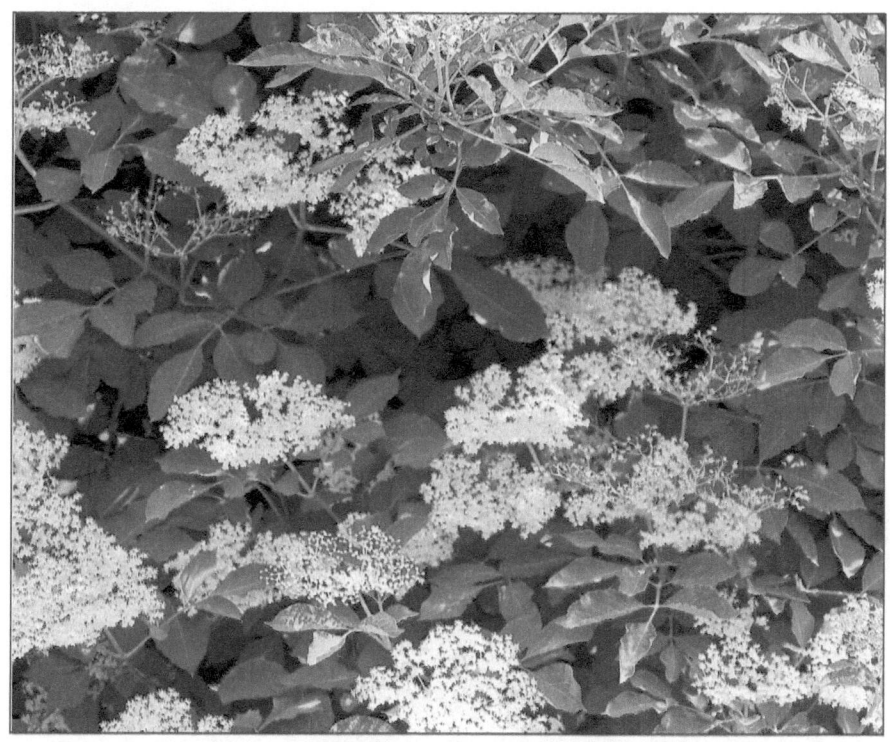

European Elder

European elder is a tree native to Europe and parts of Asia and Africa, and it also grows in the United States. The name "elder" comes from the Anglo-Saxon word "aeld," meaning fire. The terms "elder flower" and "elderberry" may refer to either European elder or a different herb called American elder. This fact sheet focuses only on European elder.

Various parts of the elder tree, including the bark, leaves, flowers, fruits, and roots, have long been used in traditional medicine.

Currently, elderberry and elder flower are used as dietary supple-ments for flu, colds, constipation, and other conditions.

The dried flowers (elder flow-er) and the dried ripe or fresh ber-ries (elderberry) of the European elder tree are used in teas, extracts, and capsules.

Although some preliminary research indicates that elderber-ry may relieve flu symptoms, the evidence is not strong enough to support its use for this purpose.

Source: https://nccih.nih.gov/health/euroelder

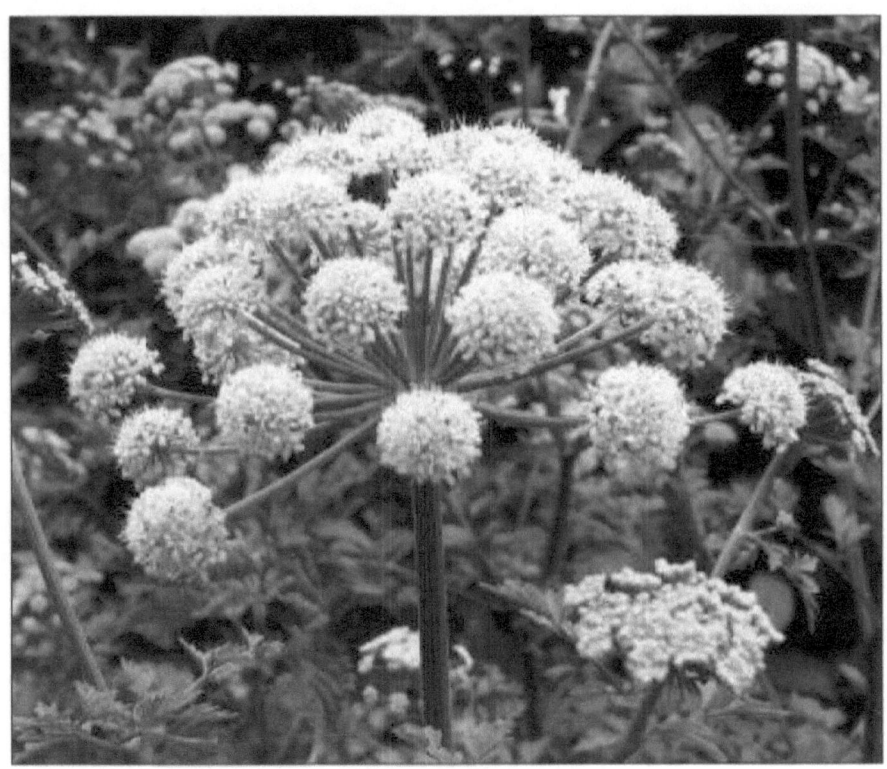

Angelica

Angelica is a very well-known medicinal plant that has been employed throughout various parts of the globe since the ancient times. Generally somewhat large, angelica species grow from between one to three metres in length depending upon the species and the viability of the environment where it thrives. They are notable for their large aromatic, bipinnate serrated leaves, but more so for their compound umbels (flower clusters) which display an often mesmerizing array of ivory-white, starK-white, or jade-white hued flowers.

Next time you have a martini, savor the flavor and remind yourself it comes from the Angelica root. Angelica herb is a European plant that has been a flavoring agent in many popular types of liquor including, gin and vermouth. The Angelica plant has a long history of use as a seasoning, medicinal and tea.

Source: https://www.gardeningknow-how.com/edible/herbs/angelica/grow-ing-angelica-herb.htm

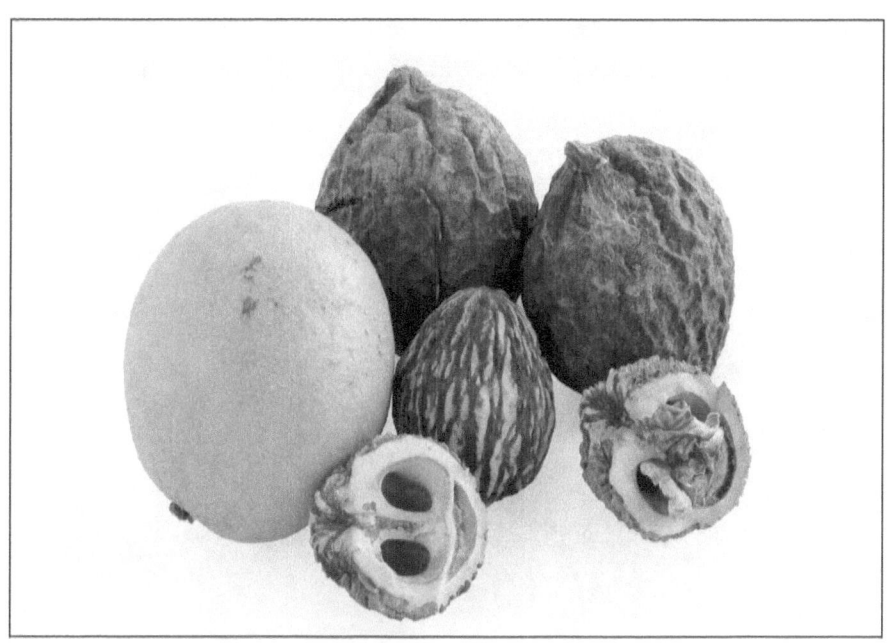

Black Walnut

Herbalists are most interested in the bark, leaves and nut husks of black walnut. Black walnut hulls contain juglone, a chemical that is antibacterial, antiviral, antiparasitic, and a fungicide. Black walnut is used to treat ringworm, yeast and candida infections. (Duke, James, Ph.D., 43) Use black walnut tea externally as a skin wash , or add the powered hulls to personal dusting powders.

Black walnut hull extract is unquestionably one of the best and safest worming agents offered by the plant world. But it can be toxic if not used with proper care, caution, and training. It is an herb best reserved for use by experienced practitioners.

Walnuts are a good dietary source of serotonin, which is important in maintaining a healthy emotional balance. A lack of serotonin in the brain is thought to be a cause of depression. Walnuts are also one of the best plant based sources of omega-3 fatty acids. Both research and population studies have shown that having the right balance of omega-3 fatty acids in the diet reduces inflammation and may help lower risk such as heart disease, cancer, and auto-immune disorders such as rheumatoid arthritis.

Source: http://www.anniesremedy.com/herb_detail221.php?gc=221&gclid=-CLH3mYTu49ICFZeNswode68EcA

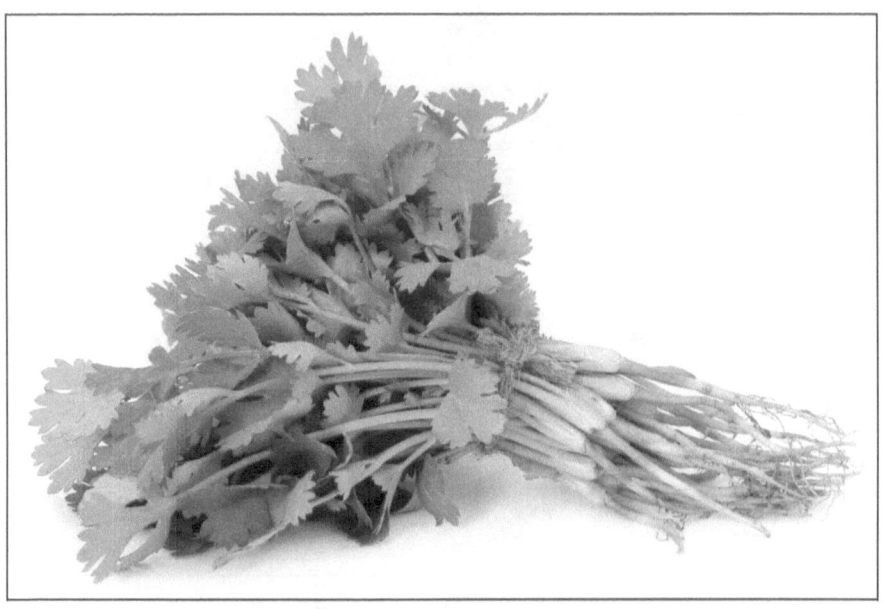

Cilantro (Coriander Leaves)

The health benefits of coriander include its use in the treatment of skin inflammation, high cholesterol levels, diarrhea, mouth ulcers, anemia, indigestion, menstrual disorders, smallpox, conjunctivitis, skin disorders, and blood sugar disorders, while also benefiting eye care.

Coriander, commonly known as Dhania in the Indian Subcontinent and Cilantro in the America and some parts of Europe, is an herb that is extensively used around the world as a condiment, garnish, or decoration on culinary dishes. Its scientific name is Coriandrum Sativum L. Its leaves and fruits have a recognizable and pleasant aroma and are common-ly used raw or dried for culinary applications.

Its uses in global food preparation is only the tip of the iceberg. Unbeknownst to many people, coriander is packed with potential health benefits that most people completely miss when they toss this garnish into the garbage after eating their meal. It has eleven components of essential oils, six types of acids (including ascorbic acid, better known as vitamin C), minerals and vitamins, each having a number of beneficial properties.

Source: https://www.organicfacts.net/ health-benefits/herbs-and-spices/ health-benefits-of-coriander.html

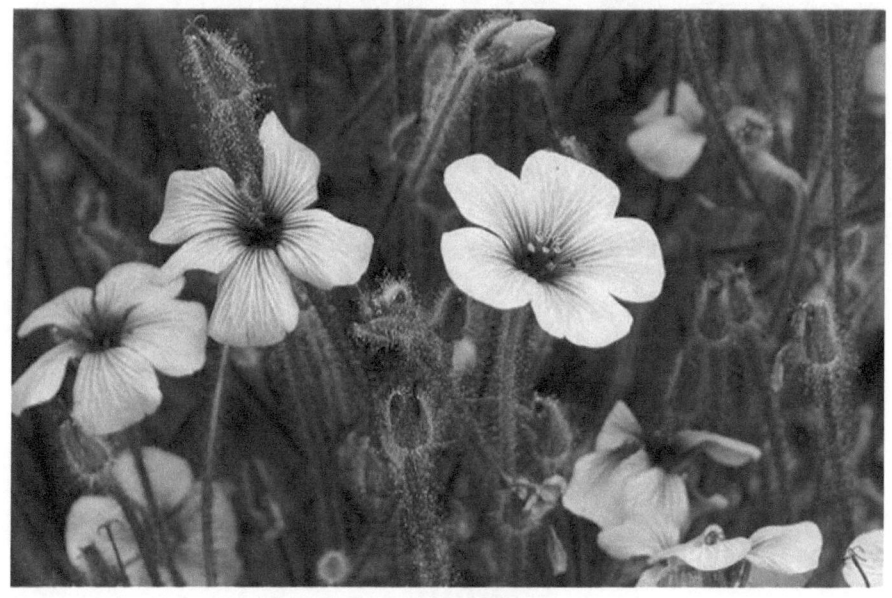

Cranesbill

Early European settlers in North America adopted this herbal medication from the indigenous Indians, as it was established that the remedy was not only effectual, but also safe. Members of the Chippewas tribe in North America dried and pounded the rhizome or the subversive stem of cranesbill to powder and applied it to lesions in the mouth, particularly in the case of kids. Other native Indian tribes suffused cranesbill in water and used the solution as eyewash. Powdered rhizome of the herb blended with different other herbs plus water was applied topically to lesions and open wounds. This blend was also used in the form of a poultice to heal swollen feet. In addition, many native Indians in North America also consumed the tender leaves of cranesbill as food.

Cranesbill is an astringent as well as a blood coagulation agent and till date the herb is being used for these properties as it was used in ancient times. Generally, herbalists prescribe cranesbill to cure irritable bowel syndrome (IBS) as well as hemorrhoids. In addition, the herb is used to heal wounds. This herb may also be employed to cure profuse menstrual bleeding as well as extreme vaginal discharges.)

Source: http://www.herbs2000.com/herbs/herbs_cranesbill.htm. A practical guide for nutritional and traditional health care.

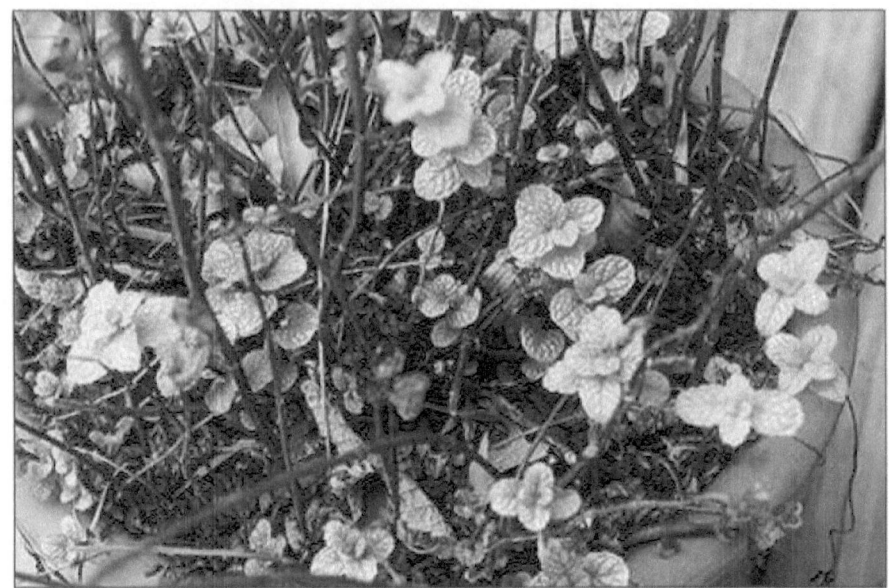

Mint

A true botanical wonder, mint is a breeze to care for, and its pleasing aroma makes it a welcome addition to the garden. The best part about this easy-to-grow herb is its usefulness. Mint makes a delicious addition to meals, a healthful tea, a fragrant potpourri and an insect-deterring spray. This sweet-smelling plant also has soothing and anesthetic properties that make it a great fit for homemade body-care products.

To grow mint, get a cutting from a friend or purchase a starter plant at a nursery. (Mint doesn't reproduce true from seed.) Mint can actually be too easy to grow—it sometimes takes over the garden—so give this attractive ground cover plenty of room to spread, or plant it in a container.

Growing mint will keep your yard and garden buzzing with beneficial insects. Mint is rich in nectar and pollen, and its small flower clusters keep these sweet treats easily accessible for helpful bugs such as honeybees and hoverflies.

While it attracts "good bugs," mint also deters "bad bugs." Repel ants and flies by growing pennyroyal mint right outside your door, or spray diluted peppermint essential oil (10 parts water to one part oil) around doorways and windows.

Source: http://www.motherearthliving.com/healthy-home/natural-cleaning/15-uses-for-mint-zmhz13mazmel

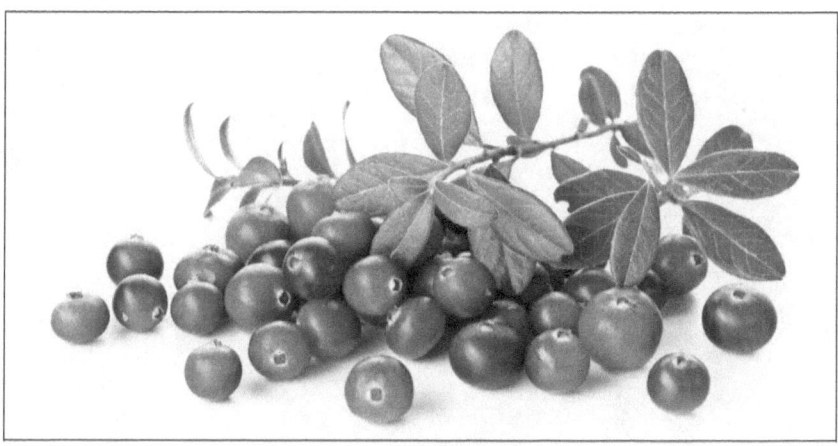

Cranberry

It is believed that the pilgrims in America enjoyed eating dishes prepared with cranberry during their maiden Thanksgiving in 1621. Gradually, this type of cranberry dishes turned out to be a national custom in the United States. However, this happened only following General Ulysses S. Grant ordering that these dishes be served to the Union troops during the American Civil War.

Native tribes in America employed cranberries in the form of a dye. A cocktail prepared with cranberry juice is also commercially available. As pure cranberry juice is very sour or acidic in taste, the cocktail is prepared by adding sugar and water to it.

In the 1840s, German researchers found out that the urine of individuals who have consumed cranberries contains hippuric acid, a chemical that combats bacteria.

Studies undertaken in recent times endorse the theory that consuming cranberries or drinking the juice of these berries may help in avoiding or combating urinary tract infections. In effect, hippuric acid thwarts the bacterium Escherichia coli (E. coli) from sticking to the lining of the urinary tract. In addition to hippuric acid, cranberry also encloses other chemical substances, such as arbutin that facilitates in combating yeast infections. Some people also use these berries in the form of a 'urinary deodorant'. Indigenous tribes of North America are believed to have prepared poultices with cranberries to heal their wounds. Thus, the American pilgrims who employed cranberries to cure fevers were not wrong or mistaken. In fact, these berries contain a high amount of vitamin C too.

Source: http://www.herbs2000.com/herbs/herbs_cranberry.htm

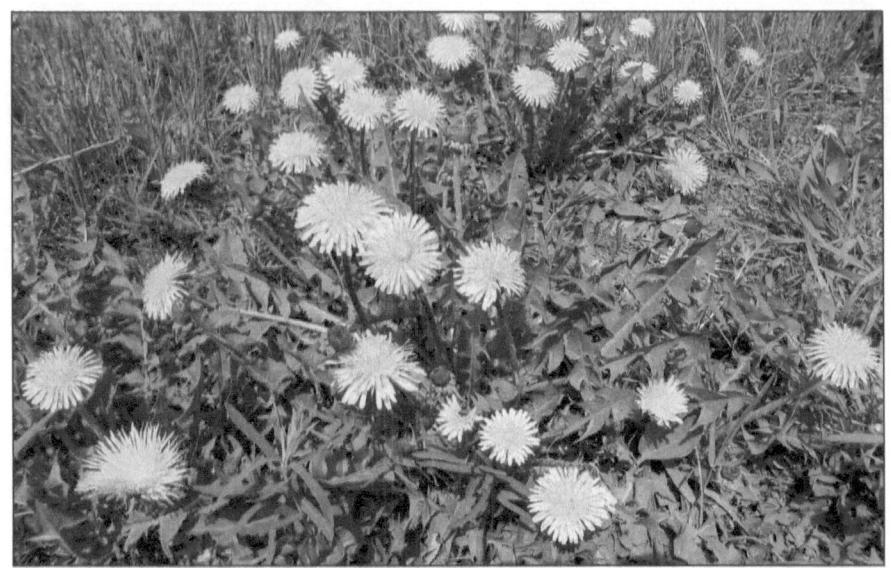

Dandelion

Dandelion greens are edible and are a rich source of vitamin A. Dandelion has been used in traditional medical systems, including Native American, traditional Chinese, and traditional Arabic medicine.

Dandelion has a long history of use for problems of the liver, gallbladder, and bile ducts. Today, dandelion as a dietary supplement is used as a blood "tonic," as a diuretic, for minor digestive problems, and for other purposes.

The leaves and roots of the dandelion, or the whole plant, are used fresh or dried in capsules or extracts. As a food, dandelion is used as a salad green and in soups, wine, and teas.[1]

Dandelion juice can help diabetic patients by stimulating the production of insulin from the pancreas, thereby keeping the blood sugar level low. Since dandelions are diuretic in nature, they increase urination in diabetic patients, which helps remove the excess sugar from the body.

Consistently lower blood sugar and a more regulated system of insulin release prevents dangerous spikes and plunges for diabetic patients, so dandelion extracts can be a perfect solution![2]

[1] Source: https://nccih.nih.gov/health/dandelion

[2] Source: https://www.organicfacts.net/health-benefits/herbs-and-spices/health-benefits-of-dandelion.html

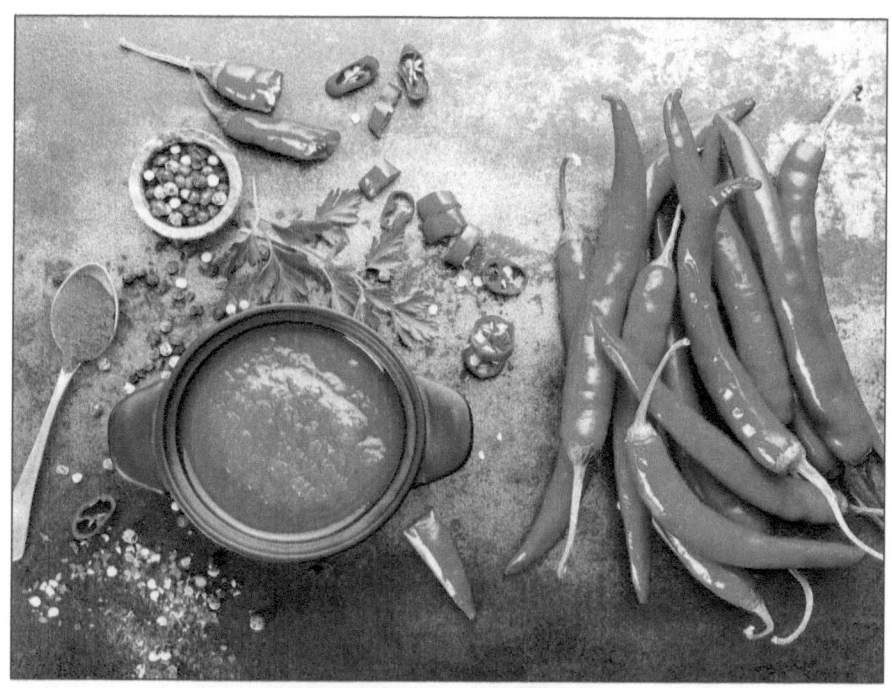

Cayenne Pepper

Many societies, especially those of the Americas and China, have a history of using cayenne pepper therapeutically. A powerful compound with many uses, cayenne pepper is currently gaining buzz for cleansing and detoxifying regimes such as the Master Cleanse, which uses the spice to stimulate circulation and neutralize acidity.

Cayenne pepper has been used for a variety of ailments including heartburn, delirium, tremors, gout, paralysis, fever, dyspepsia, atonic dyspepsia, flatulence, sore throat, hemorrhoids, menorrhagia in women, nausea, tonsillitis, scarlet fever, and diphtheria. Let's take a look at just two of the best health benefits cayenne pepper has to offer:

• Cayenne has the ability to ease upset stomach, ulcers, sore throats, spasmodic and irritating coughs, and diarrhea.

• Suffering from stuffed up sinuses due to cold, flu, or allergies? Cayenne pepper aids in breaking up and moving congested mucus.

Source: http://www.globalhealingcenter.com/natural-health/benefits-of-cayenne-pepper/ (by Dr. Edward Group DC, NP, DACBN, DCBCN, DABFM, Published on June 21, 2010, Last Updated on October 21, 2015)

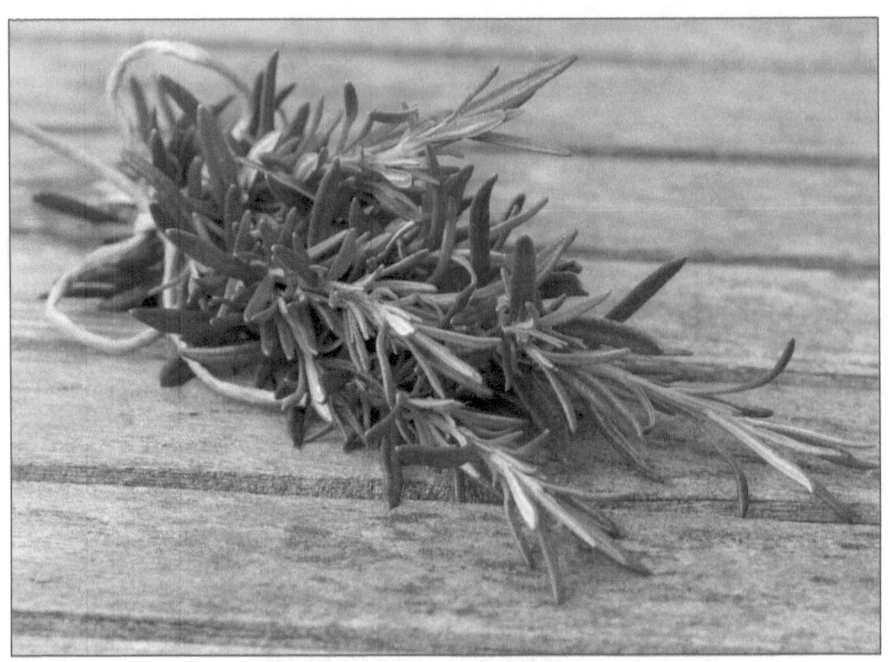

Rosemary

Rosemary Leaf is an aromatic herb in the mint family that grows on an evergreen bush. It is most often used in cooking but has a wonderful woodsy scent that is great in air fresheners and aromatherapy mixes.

Concentrated extracts like Rosemary Oil should be used externally, although the dried herb can be taken internally when used in cooking. It is an especially great herb to add to meats (and pairs well with lamb). Some research suggests that it has anti-cancer properties.

Rosemary can be infused into an oil and used externally for skin irritations like eczema and joint problems like arthritis

It has also been reported to speed healing of wounds and bruises when used externally

Internally, it is best added to foods as a cooking spice, though a mild tea of Rosemary Leaf can help fight illness when sipped

A strong infusion of Rosemary and Nettle leaf is an excellent herbal rinse for hair and can help get rid of dandruff and speed hair growth when used after each washing

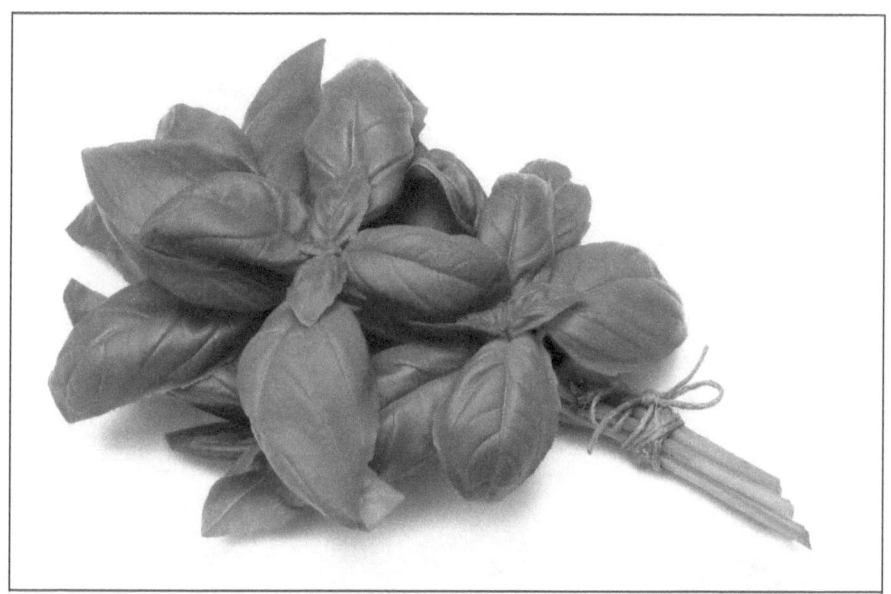

Sweet Basil

Basil is most known for its culinary uses. What isn't as well known are the various other herbal uses of Basil. It is a traditional remedy that has been used in various cultures for hundreds of years for many uses besides cooking. These are some top uses:

Basil Pesto – This culinary use is one of Basil's most popular uses and variations of this are used in cultures around the world. Add pesto to everything from eggs, to meats, to slices of fresh cucumber.

General Cooking – Dried basil can be easily added to practically any dish. Basil is used around the world in many different cuisines with good reason. It adds a depth and flavor that is not rivaled by other herbs. Make a homemade spice blend that includes basil and add it to practically anything.

Calming the Stomach – The Italians may be on to something with adding Basil to everything. It is thought to have a calming effect on the stomach and 1/2 teaspoon of dried or fresh basil leaf in water can often help sooth indigestion and alleviate feelings of fullness.

Try using Basil leaf to help alleviate coughing and colds. Chew fresh leaves to calm coughing or make a calming tea of dried basil to help sooth illness.

Source: https://wellnessmama.com/5505/uses-for-basil-leaf/

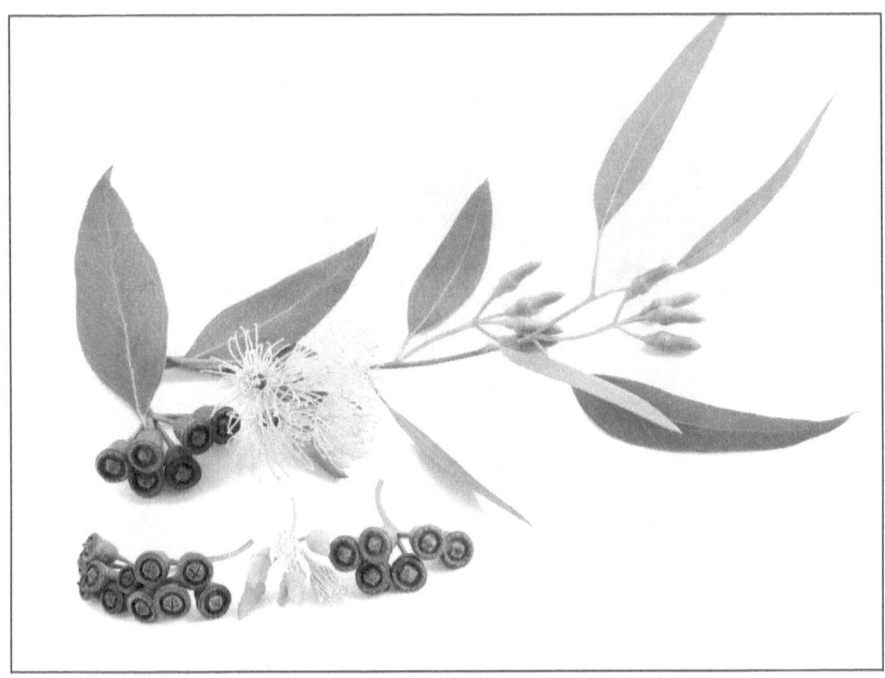

Eucalyptus

The eucalyptus tree is an evergreen tree native to Australia that's often thought of as the main food source of koala bears. While it provides amazing nutritional support for wildlife, the essential oils extracted from eucalyptus leaves also have powerful medicinal properties.

According to English folklore, an early English settler had his thumb nearly severed by an ax. His father, who was well-versed in Aboriginal folk medicine, advised that he apply a bandage of tightly bound eucalyptus leaves around the cut after it was sutured.

Later, when a surgeon saw the wound, he remarked how amazed he was because the thumb healed so quickly and without any trace of infection.

Interestingly, small towns in Australia discovered that eucalyptus oil could be converted into a gas to light their homes, hotels and shops. Little did they know that they stumbled upon one of the most powerful forms of natural medicine ever.

Today, eucalyptus oil uses have a broad range of health benefits.

Source: https://draxe.com/eucalyptus-oil-uses-benefits/

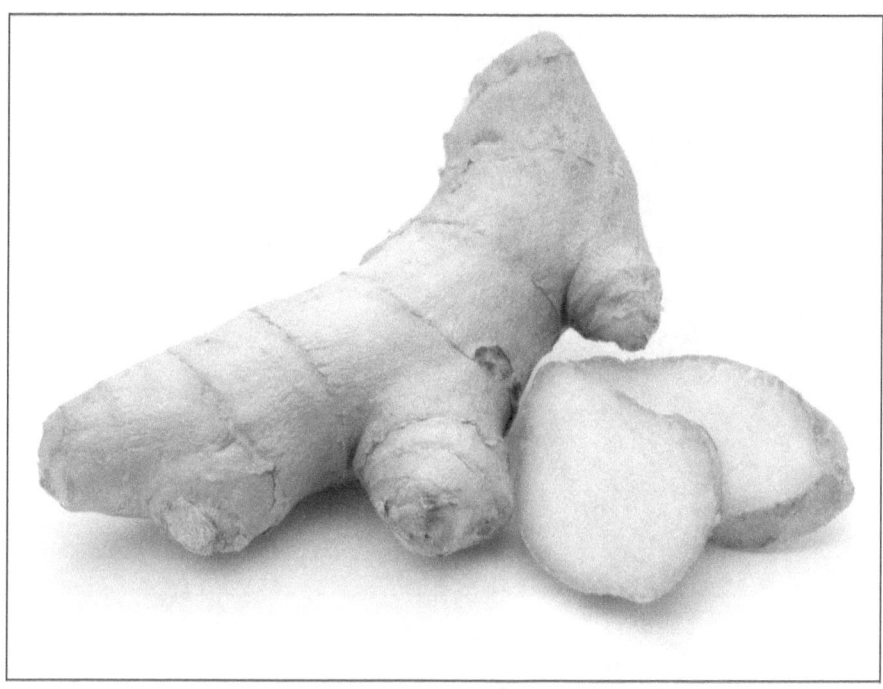

Ginger Root

Ginger is among the healthiest (and most delicious) spices on the planet. It is loaded with nutrients and bioactive compounds that have powerful benefits for your body and brain.

Ginger is a popular spice. It is high in gingerol, a substance with powerful anti-inflammatory and antioxidant properties. 1-1.5 grams of ginger can help prevent various types of nausea. This applies to sea sickness, chemotherapy-related nausea, nausea after surgery and morning sickness.

Ginger appears to be effective at reducing the day-to-day progression of muscle pain, and may reduce exercise-induced muscle soreness. There are some studies showing ginger to be effective at reducing symptoms of osteoarthritis, which is a very common health problem.

Ginger has been shown to lower blood sugar levels and improve various heart disease risk factors in patients with type 2 diabetes

Ginger appears to speed up emptying of the stomach, which can be beneficial for people with indigestion and related stomach discomfort.

Source: https://authoritynutrition.com/11-proven-benefits-of-ginger/

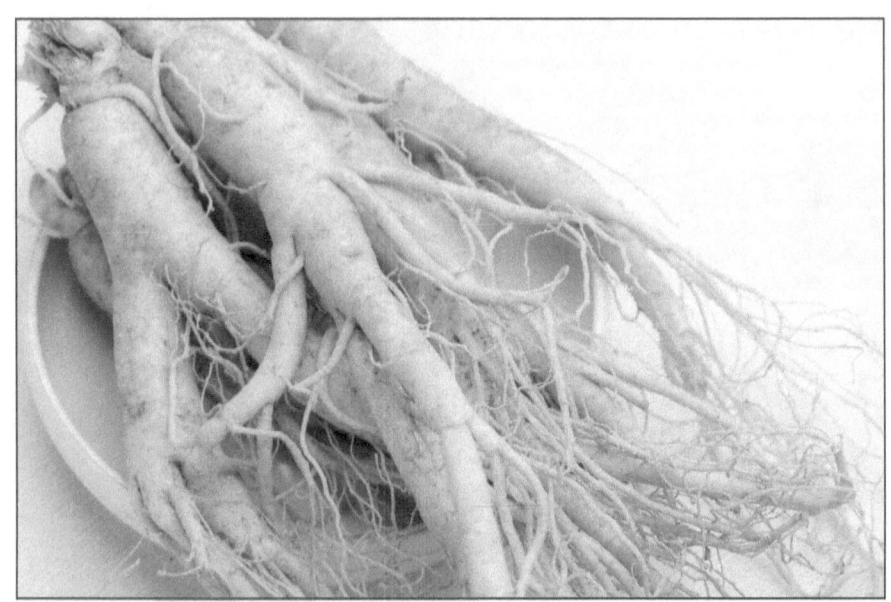

Ginseng

Ginseng is one of the most popular herbal supplements in the US, perhaps most well known for its traditional use of boosting memory and energy levels. However, it has many other uses. For starters, ginseng is considered an adaptogen, which means it helps your body to withstand mental and physical stress.

Most research to date has involved Asian ginseng, however the studies that have been done on the American variety suggest it may boost your immune system, function as an antioxidant and also benefit inflammatory conditions. It may also be useful as an all-around stress tonic. According to research published in the Journal of Herbs, Spices & Medicinal Plants.

If you're wondering which type of ginseng is right for you, consider this: if you're seeking an herb to calm stress-related problems, American ginseng is the "cooling" or "calming" version of the two. Asian ginseng is regarded as heating and is not generally recommended for stress relief.

Ginseng shows promise for protecting heart health, including anti-hypertensive effects and protection against heart failure. Asian ginseng, in particular, may protect against symptoms of heart disease and support healthy cholesterol levels.

Source: http://articles.mercola.com/sites/articles/archive/2015/06/22/ginseng-health-benefits.aspx

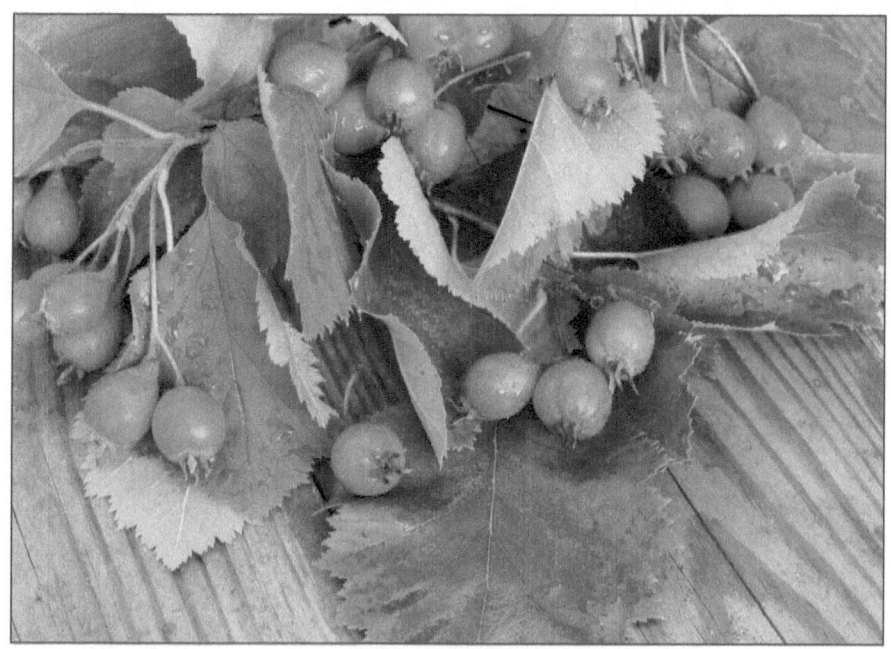

Hawthorn Berries

A dense bush bearing tiny red berries, hawthorn bushes are common in wooded areas and fence rows across the U.S. and throughout the world. Many parts of the hawthorn (with the botanical name Crataegus), including its berries and flowers, have been used by traditional healers for centuries.

Resembling tiny sweet cherries, hawthorn berry "haws" have been used to make wine, jelly and flavored brandy for years, but not many people are aware of the impressive ways it remedies heart problems and many other physical ailments as well.

Increasingly, modern studies are pointing to the hawthorn plant as a valuable therapy for cardiovascular disease (CVD), which the U.S. Centers for Disease Control and Prevention (CDC) states is the most prevalent cause of death in the U.S. In fact, more than 2.6 million people died of it in 2015.

The hawthorn berry bush belongs to the same family of plants as apples and roses, so it's fitting that the fruit is usually brilliant red. Like roses on steroids, the berries are accompanied by long, woody thorns that can do a lot of damage if you're not cautious.

Source: http://articles.mercola.com/sites/articles/archive/2016/10/24/hawthorn-berry-benefits.aspx

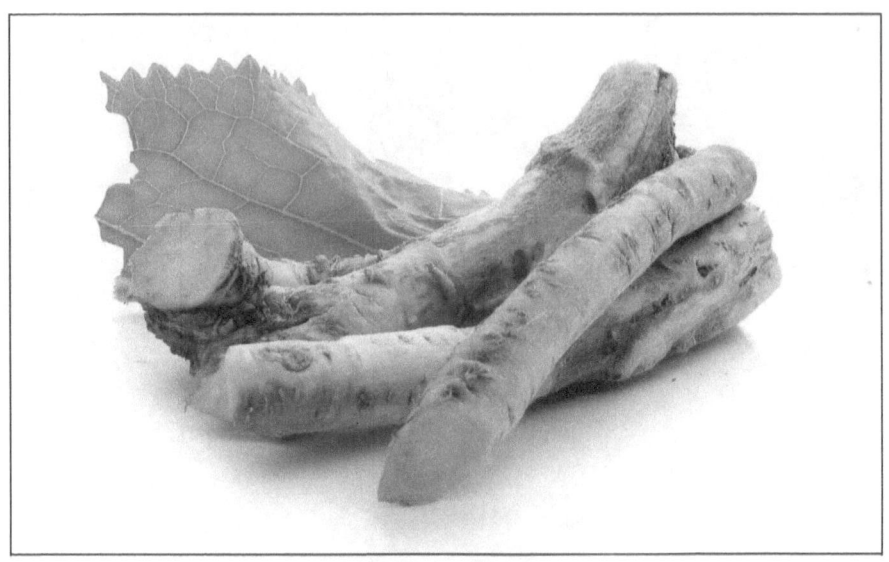

Horseradish

Horseradish is a powerful and pungent plant that is connected to a wide variety of health benefits, including its ability to aid weight loss, lower blood pressure, alleviate respiratory conditions, build strong bones, improve immune system health, stimulate healthy digestion, promote heart health, and lower the chances of neural tube defects in infants.

Horseradish is very low in calories, only 6 per serving, and has no fat whatsoever. It does have omega-3 and omega-6 fatty acids but they are an essential part of human metabolism, so just because they are labeled as "cholesterol" doesn't mean that consuming them is always bad. Since it is high in fiber and rich in protein, horseradish can stimulate feelings of satiety, and it can be used freely in recipes without worrying about adding any unnecessary fats or calories.

Potassium is an essential part of our bodies that regulates the flow of cellular fluids and regulates the tension of blood vessels. Potassium deficiency results in higher blood pressure, which means a higher risk of contracting cardiovascular diseases and conditions like atherosclerosis, heart attacks, and strokes. Eating horseradish, which is a rich source of potassium, can increase your heart health by lowering your blood pressure and regulating the passage of fluids and nutrients between cellular membranes.

Source: https://www.organicfacts.net/health-benefits/vegetable/horseradish.html

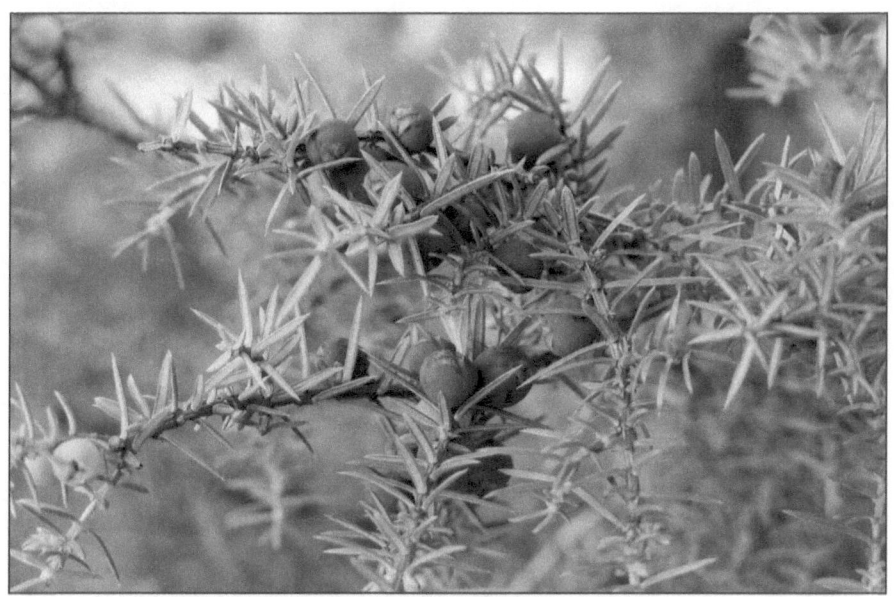

Juniper with Berries

Juniper is native to the northern hemisphere and is common in Canada, Scandinavia and Siberia. It is is an erect evergreen coniferous shrub or a small tree which can grow up to ten meters tall.

Juniper has been used traditionally to treat arthritis, gout and rheumatism. Test tube studies have shown that the berries can inhibit prostaglandin synthesis which indicates that this traditional use has some merit.

Juniper has diuretic and antiseptic properties which explains its uses as an herbal remedy for urinary tract infections such as cystitis and urethritis. Modern studies on juniper indicate that it increases the filtration rate of the kidneys, dilutes the urine and disinfects the urinary tract.

Other traditional medical uses for juniper berries are the treatment of intestinal infections, colic and other stomach upsets. Additionally it has been used as a medicinal herb for coughs, bronchitis and upper respiratory infections. In the German Pharmacopoeia the berries are listed as a treatment for dyspeptic complaints such as gas, heartburn, indigestion and flatulence.

The herb has been used topically as a treatment for wounds, muscle aches, lesions and abnormal skin growths, and snake bites.

Source: https://www.herbal-supplement-resource.com/juniper-herb.html

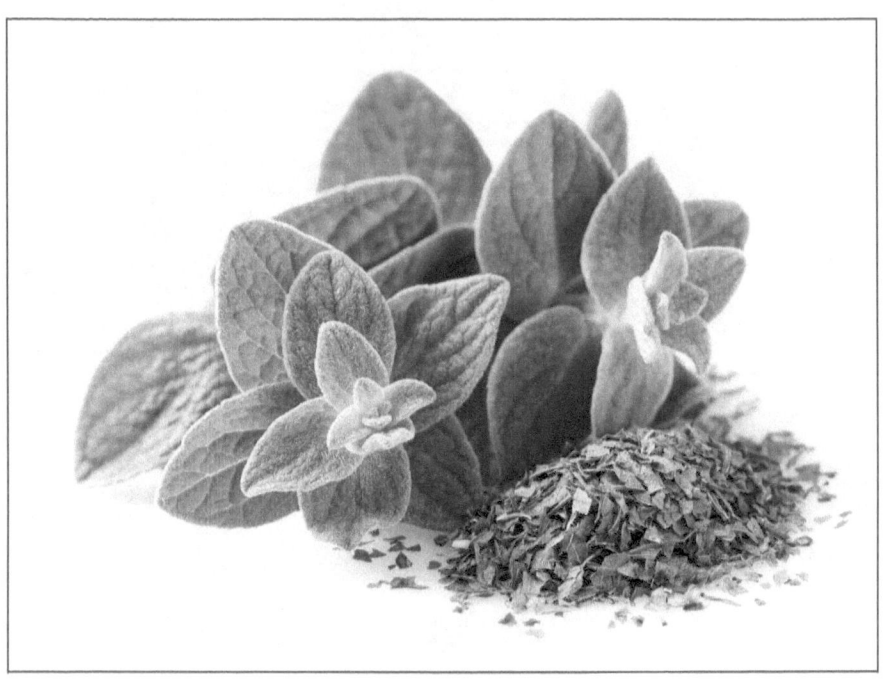

Oregano

Oregano is an important culinary and medicinal herb that has been used in medicine and cooking for thousands of years - with a number of potential health benefits.

Not only does oregano provide food flavor, there are also a substantial number of health claims associated with its potent antioxidants and anti-bacterial properties.

Oregano has a very pleasant aromatic scent. The herb is used to treat respiratory tract disorders, gastrointestinal (GI) disorders, menstrual cramps, and urinary tract disorders.

The herb is also applied topically to help treat a number of skin conditions, such as acne and dandruff.

Oregano contains fiber, iron, manganese, vitamin E, iron, calcium, omega fatty acids, manganese, and typtophan.

Oregano is also a rich source of Vitamin K, an important vitamin which promotes bone growth, the maintenance of bone density, and the production of blood clotting proteins.

Source: http://www.medicalnewstoday.com/articles/266259.php

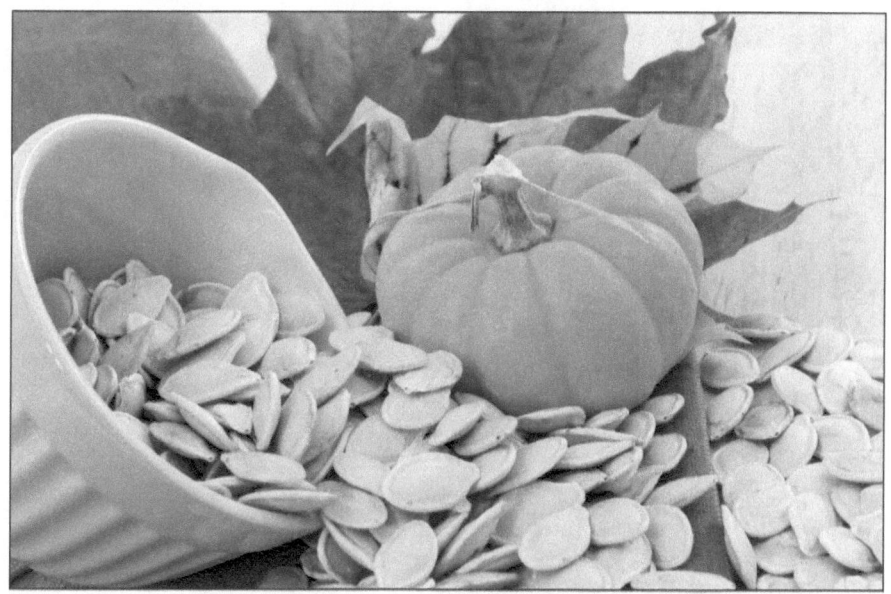

Pumpkin Seeds

Along with being a great tasting culinary oil, pumpkin oil is most commonly taken for preventing hair loss and prostate problems, due to its reported DHT blocking properties.

Like the seeds, raw pumpkin seed oil can help improve skin tone and may be a beneficial supplement for many skin problems like acne, dry flaky skin, eczema and psoriasis. Alongside the powerful antioxidant content, the high levels of natural fats would appear to be responsible for this effect.

The fatty acids in this healthy oil assist in maintaining smooth skin tone and will help speed up the repair of dry, flaky and irritated skin. They are also important for proper moisture levels within the epidermis and normalizing skin's oil production.

Pumpkin seed oil has also being used as a treatment for irritable bowel syndrome, for dealing with intestinal parasites like tapeworms, to lessen the symptoms of osteoporosis and to prevent and even treat kidney stone problems.

Pumpkin seed oil has also being used as a treatment for irritable bowel syndrome, for dealing with intestinal parasites like tapeworms, to lessen the symptoms of osteoporosis and to prevent and even treat kidney stone problems.

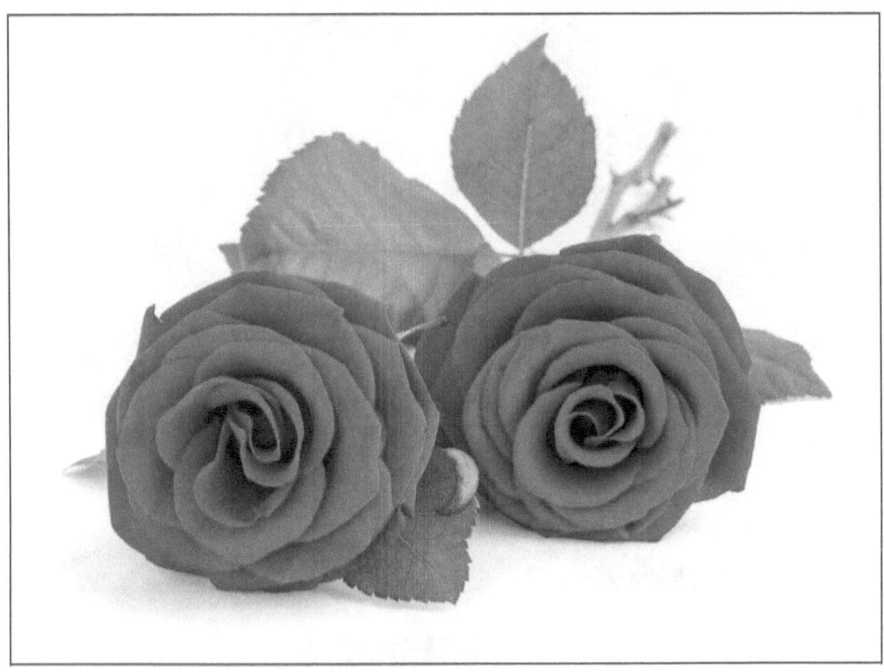

Rose

A rose is a woody, thorny plant of the rosaceae family. There are more than one hundred species of roses, with large showy flowers in many different colors. Roses are considered native to Asia, but are also grown in Europe, northern Africa, and North America.

"A rose by any other name would smell as sweet," says Juliet in Shakespeare's Romeo and Juliet, which is so very true of the rose that has captured the minds and hearts of people through the ages. The rose, however, has proved its veritable worth owing to its exhaustive use in health and medicine.

The medicinal uses and health benefits of a rose (gulab flower) are many. Rose petals are used in making rose oil that is steam distilled by crushing. The byproduct of steam distillation is rose water, which is an excellent relaxing agent, soothes the nerves and adds flavor to a variety of dishes across the world. Rose essence is rich in flavanoids, tannins, antioxidants, and vitamins A, B3, C, D and E, making it beneficial in skin care.

Source: http://www.diethealthclub.com/health-food/rose-health-benefits.html

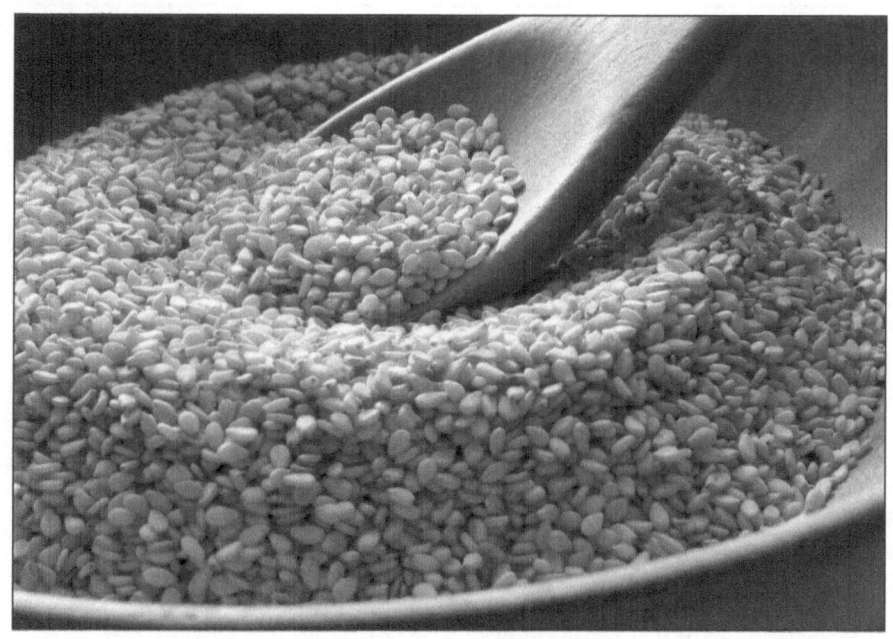

Sesame Seeds

Sesame seeds may be the oldest condiment known to man. They are highly valued for their oil which is exceptionally resistant to rancidity. "Open sesame"—the famous phrase from the Arabian Nights—reflects the distinguishing feature of the sesame seed pod, which bursts open when it reaches maturity.

Sesame seeds add a nutty taste and a delicate, almost invisible, crunch to many Asian dishes. They are also the main ingredients in tahini (sesame seed paste) and the wonderful Middle Eastern sweet call halvah.

Not only are sesame seeds an excellent source of copper and a very good source of manganese, but they are also a good source of calcium, magnesium, iron, phosphorus, vitamin B1, zinc, molybdenum, selenium, and dietary fiber. In addition to these important nutrients, sesame seeds contain two unique substances: sesamin and sesamolin. Both of these substances belong to a group of special beneficial fibers called lignans, and have been shown to have a cholesterol-lowering effect in humans, and to prevent high blood pressure and increase vitamin E supplies in animals.

Source: http://www.whfoods.com/gen-page.php?tname=foodspice&dbid=84

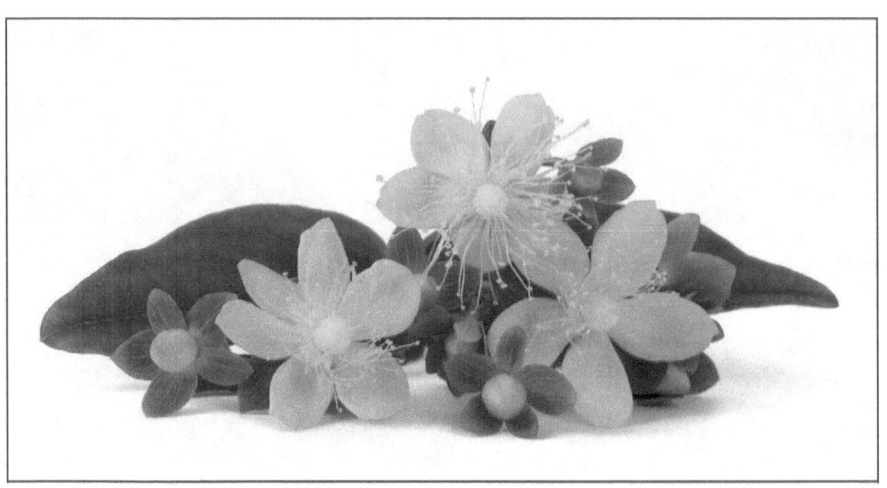

St. John's Wort

St. John's wort, also known as hypericum perforatum, is a flowering plant of the genus Hypericum and has been used as a medicinal herb for its antidepressant and anti-inflammatory properties for over 2,000 years. The Greek physicians of the first century recommended the use of St. John's wort for its medicinal value, and the ancients believed that the plant had mystical and protective qualities.

Dating back to the ancient Greeks, St. John's wort uses included treatment for illnesses such as various nervous or mood disorders. Scientists believe it's native to Europe, parts of Asia and Africa, and the Western United States. St. John's wort was given its name because it blooms around June 24, the birthday of John the Baptist, and the word "wort" is an old English word for plant.

St. John's wort is most commonly used to naturally remedy depression and symptoms, such as anxiety, tiredness, loss of appetite and trouble sleeping. It's also used to treat heart palpitations, moodiness, the symptoms of attention deficit-hyperactivity disorder (ADHD), obsessive-compulsive disorder (OCD), seasonal affective disorder (SAD) and symptoms of menopause.

A native to Europe, St. John's wort is also commonly found in the United States and Canada in the dry ground of roadsides, meadows and woods. Although not native to Australia and long considered a weed, St. John's wort is now grown there as a crop, and today Australia produces 20 percent of the world's supply

Source: https://draxe.com/st-johns-wort-uses/

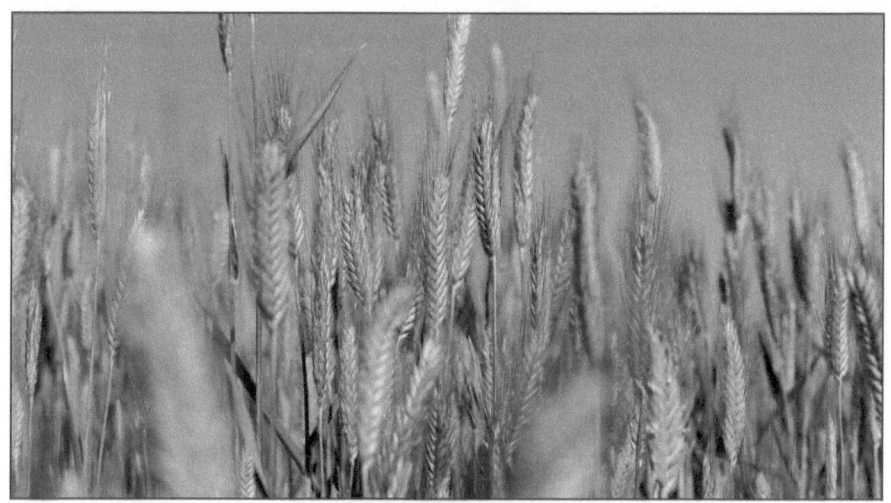

Wheatgrass

If you haven't jumped on the wheatgrass bandwagon yet, it's not too late. Yes, OK, wheatgrass can seem like the kind of health trend you chalk up to hipsters, treehuggers, and more-or-less-obsessed health and fitness enthusiasts, but if folks are wheatgrass obsessed, it's for good reason: wheatgrass juice is perhaps the healthiest food out there, and wheatgrass benefits run the gamut, from increased energy levels to improved overall health to head-to-toe beauty.

Still not convinced? Maybe these 35 reasons why wheatgrass need to become part of your daily routine will change your tune.

Wheatgrass boasts some impressive nutritional stats. It's an excellent source of chlorophyll, vitamin A, vitamin C, and vitamin E, and to top it all off wheatgrass contains 98 of 102 earth elements found in soil, including phosphorus, calcium, iron, magnesium, and potassium as well as essential enzymes and 19 amino acids. Wheatgrass is also overflowing with vitamins, and liver enzymes.

The star of wheatgrass' nutritional makeup is chlorophyll, a phytochemical that gives dark leafy greens their color. Chlorophyll is essentially the blood of plants; and in humans, it reverses aging, suppresses hunger, cleanses the blood, combats odor, and has been linked to the prevention of cancer. Wheatgrass is made up of 70 percent chlorophyll — it's no wonder it's so powerful.

Source: http://www.organicauthority.com/benefits-of-wheatgrass.html

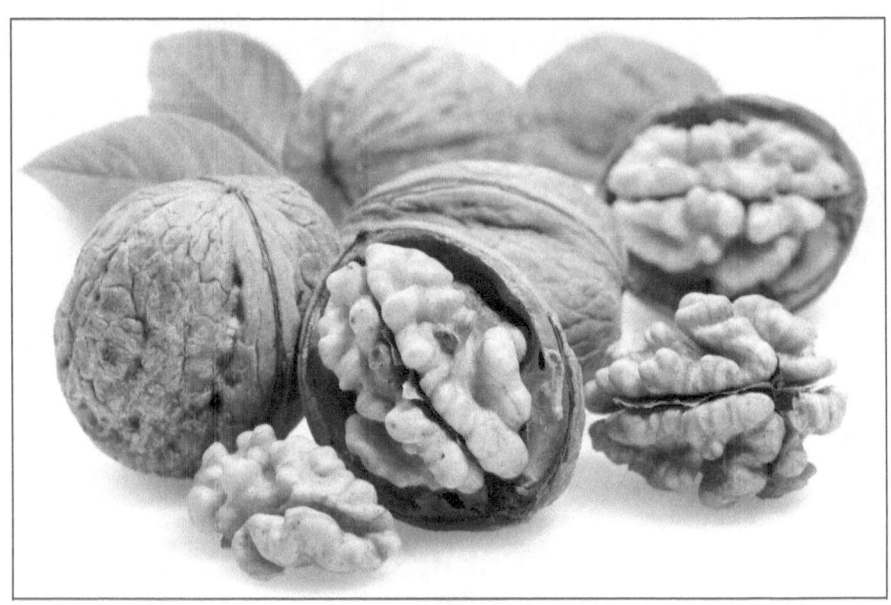

Walnut

Walnuts are actually seeds not nuts! They grow in little green fruits that look like grainy textured apples on walnut trees, which are any tree from the genus Juglans. Once the green skin is peeled off, a more familiar sight is seen. The hard shell is difficult to crack open, but inside is one of most popular nuts in the world. It is shaped like a brain, but studies show it heals the heart.

The best thing about walnuts is that they are one of the healthiest foods that are cultivated to be eaten. Studies promote them as a perfect dietary supplement. This is especially true because of the wide range of benefits they provide for physical health. They have preventive properties to keep fitness in check.

Walnuts can be eaten raw or roasted. Neither preparation will diminish their nutritive value. The area of the body that receives the most help from walnuts is the heart and the rest of the circulatory system. They lower the risk of blood clotting by ensuring that blood vessels are clean and clear. They also keep blood pressure steady. Studies show that the nutrients present in walnuts optimize the circulatory system into a well-balanced and efficiently functioning unit. The omega-3 in walnuts helps in this.

Source: http://www.herbwisdom.com/herb-walnuts.html

www.ingramcontent.com/pod-product-compliance
Lightning Source LLC
Chambersburg PA
CBHW020905310526
45786CB00018B/1832